Yoga for Beginners

The Ultimate Guide to Poses and Practices

Table of Contents

Chapter 1. Introduction

Prepare to embark on an enlightening journey into the world of yoga in our Special Report - "Yoga for Beginners: The Ultimate Guide to Poses and Practices". This all-encompassing guide is your ticket to achieving physical wellbeing, mastering mental calm, and unlocking your true potential. Tailored specifically for novices, it breaks down complex yoga terms, poses, and practices into bite-sized, easily digestible pieces of wisdom. Whether you want to strike a Mountain Pose, take a deep dive into Pranayama, or simply wish to embrace the tranquillity yoga offers, this guide serves as your perfect stepping stone. Absorb years of yogic wisdom curated into a single comprehensive report which is as easy to understand as it is to practice. Now is your time to stretch beyond the ordinary, enhance your inner vitality, and let yoga transform your life one breath at a time. So, why wait? Grab on to this report and let your yoga journey begin!

Chapter 2. Embarking on the Yoga Journey: An Introduction

Yoga, an ancient practice with its roots anchored in India, has unequivocally stood the test of time. Its timeless wisdom holds the key to unlocking a realm of physical, mental, and spiritual well-being that is personalized to your needs and abilities.

Before you leap onto this profound path, it is paramount that you grasp the essence of yoga and its vast tapestry.

2.1. Understanding Yoga

Yoga, derived from the Sanskrit word 'Yuj,' translates to 'union' or 'to yoke.' Consider it as a holistic discipline that seeks union of the body, mind, and spirit. It incorporates a combination of physical, mental, and spiritual practices such as asanas, meditation, and ethical disciplines. More than a mere system of exercise, it is a pathway to holistic health, self-realization, and heightened awareness.

Yoga's properties are not simply confined to the physical. Yoga asanas (poses) are indeed known to enhance physical flexibility, balance, and strength, but that's merely scratching the surface. Meditation and mindful practices blended within yoga endow inner peace, mental clarity, and emotional balance, anchoring you amidst life's tumult.

2.2. Yoga Philosophy and Its Eight Limbs

At the heart of Yoga lies Patanjali's Yoga Sutras, a fundamental text delineating the philosophy and practices of yoga. An integral part of this is the concept of the 'Ashtanga' or the 'Eight-Limbed Path.'

Understanding these elements can provide you with a broader context of your practice:

1. Yama: These are ethical standards or moral disciplines, encompassing non-violence, truthfulness, non-stealing, continence, and non-greed.

2. Niyama: These involve self-discipline and spiritual observances.

3. Asana: These are the physical postures performed in yoga.

4. Pranayama: This aspect pertains to breath control and the mastery over the prana, or life force.

5. Pratyahara: Represents withdrawal or sensory transcendence, in which we disconnect from external influences and focus inward.

6. Dharana: Concentration and fostering inner perceptual awareness.

7. Dhyana: Meditation or contemplation, the uninterrupted flow of concentration.

8. Samadhi: Attaining a state of ecstasy, wherein you merge with your point of focus and transcend physical consciousness.

2.3. Navigating Through Yoga Styles

As diverse as we humans are, so too is the presentation of yoga. Numerous styles have evolved over time, each offering a unique approach. Some of the primary styles include Hatha Yoga, Vinyasa Yoga, Bikram Yoga, Iyengar Yoga, and Kundalini Yoga.

Hatha Yoga is often ideal for beginners due to its slower pace, while Vinyasa Yoga integrates fluid, movement-intensive practices. Iyengar Yoga emphasizes postural alignment and often uses props for support, while Kundalini Yoga fuses spiritual practices with physical routines. Choosing a style that resonates with your fitness goals and individual preferences can enhance your journey.

2.4. Embracing Beginner's Mind

As you embark on your yoga journey, remember to embrace a "beginner's mind." This Zen concept refers to cultivating an open mind, free from preconceptions. Beginning yoga can challenge your body and mind in unfamiliar ways. Keeping an open, curious mindset can help you adapt, understand, and commit to your ongoing self-discovery.

2.5. Yoga Sessions: What to Expect?

Typically, a yoga session initiates with a brief period of grounding or quiet time, where you relax and center your thoughts. Following this, you transition into warm-up exercises or easy postures to prepare your body. The session then evolves into more active asanas, before culminating in relaxation or meditation.

2.6. Getting Equipped: Yoga Essentials

Getting started with yoga doesn't require elaborate equipment. However, having the right gear can augment your practice. A well-cushioned yoga mat, comfortable clothing allowing easy movement, and possibly props like yoga blocks or straps for supporting certain postures, are a handy initial yoga kit.

Embarking on the journey of yoga can be transformative. It is a path that asks for discipline, perseverance, and patience but reciprocates with priceless gifts of holistic health, inner peace, and self-realization. Embrace yoga not just as an activity or routine but as a means to self-discovery, mindfulness, and wellbeing. Remain patient, and allow your journey to unfold at its own pace. Remember, yoga is not a destination but a path of self-exploration, growth, and unity.

This guide will fuel your journey, elucidating the intricacies of yoga, demystifying complex poses, and outlining how to thread yoga into your lifestyle. Pause, breathe, and let us delve deeper into the world of yoga, one pose, one breath at a time.

Chapter 3. Understanding the Fundamentals: Yoga Philosophies and Principles

Let's get started by walking into the ancient realm of Yoga. Dating back around 5,000 years, it has piqued human curiosity, enlightenment, and well-being throughout the centuries. Breathtaking in both its richness and depth, Yoga encompasses a myriad of facets that extend far beyond the physical postures we usually perceive.

3.1. Yoga: More than Just Poses

Yoga is undeniably much more than just poses (or 'asanas' as they're traditionally called). The asanas are merely one among the eight limbs of yoga elucidated in Patanjali's Yoga Sutras - an ancient, authoritative text on yogic philosophy. These eight limbs serve as a comprehensive roadmap, outlining the path from the mundane to the profound, from suffering to liberation.

To comprehend yoga in its depth, we must also delve into meditation (Dhyana), morality (Yamas and Niyamas), breath control (Pranayama), sensory withdrawal (Pratyahara), concentration (Dharana), and ultimate liberation (Samadhi).

3.2. The Foundations: Yamas and Niyamas

The Yamas and Niyamas form the moral backbone of yoga. They constitute ethical guidelines that elucidate the path of mindfulness and empathy in a person's life.

The Yamas are moral proscriptions that guide us on how to interact with the world around us. They form the basic universal morality and include five principles:

1. Ahimsa (Non-violence): Encourages kind, considerate conduct and triggers our compassion. Ahimsa urges respect for all living beings, including oneself.

2. Satya (Truthfulness): Addresses our interactions and urges honesty towards oneself and others, both in action and speech.

3. Asteya (Non-stealing): Espouses not taking anything not freely given.

4. Brahmacharya (Moderation): Promotes the control of senses and abstinence from overindulgence.

5. Aparigraha (Non-possessiveness): Inspires us to detach from material possessions and live a life free of greed.

Niyamas are the personal observances that enrich an inner spiritual life. They include:

1. Saucha (Purity): It calls for cleanliness of body, mind, and environment.

2. Santosha (Contentment): Encourages acceptance and contentment with what we have and where we are in life.

3. Tapas (Discipline): The willingness to persist and endure challenges.

4. Svadhyaya (Self-study): Encourages introspection and the study of sacred scriptures.

5. Ishvara Pranidhana (Surrender to the divine): The act of surrendering and dedicating oneself to the divine or a higher power.

3.3. Asanas: The Physical Aspect of Yoga

Asanas form the physical practice of yoga. Despite being only a part of yoga, the biomechanics and benefits of asanas are immense. They improve strength and flexibility, enhance blood circulation, and lower stress levels.

Each asana has specific benefits attached to it. For instance, the Balasana (Child's pose) calms the mind while gently stretching the hips and thighs; the Tadasana (Mountain pose) improves posture and balance; the Savasana (Corpse pose) induces total body-and-mind relaxation.

3.4. Pranayama: The Breath of Life

Pranayama is the practice of breath control in yoga. 'Prana' means 'life force', 'yama' means 'control', thus Pranayama is essentially the control of the life force.

Every yogic breath brings with it a host of benefits – from stress reduction to improved digestion; increased mental clarity to enhanced lung capacity. Different Pranayama techniques such as Anulom-vilom (Alternate Nostril Breathing), Kapalbhati (Skull Shining Breath), Bhramari (Bee Breath), etc., are designed to rejuvenate different aspects of our being.

3.5. Dharana, Dhyana, and Samadhi: The Spiritual Aspects of Yoga

These final three steps of yoga lead the practitioner to spiritual enlightenment. Dharana means concentration or focus, Dhyana refers to contemplation or meditation, and Samadhi refers to an ecstatic union with the divine.

Dharana involves stilling the mind by focusing on a single point. Dhyana is deep meditation, which builds upon Dharana's focus. Samadhi is the state of oneness achieved through profound meditation, where the meditator, the process of meditation, and the object of meditation merge into one.

From ethical living to divine realization, Yoga is a comprehensive lifestyle approach that promotes overall physical, mental, and spiritual health. As we've unveiled in this chapter, there's much more to yoga than the physical postures we often associate it with. To truly harness yoga's transformative power, we must incorporate its multi-faceted principles and practices into our lives.

Chapter 4. Gear Up: Essential Tools for Your Practice

Before you embark on your transformative journey into the realm of yoga, it's crucial to ensure you have the essential tools and gear necessary to guide your practice. Gathering these items beforehand will enable a seamless transition into yoga and its practices, making your experience far more pleasant and encouraging.

4.1. The Yoga Mat

No tool is as pivotal to your yoga experience as the yoga mat. It serves as your sacred space, a place where you surrender your distractions and immerse yourself in the serenity of the present moment. The mat observes all your poses, breaths, and movements, absorbing the energy of your concentrated efforts.

While yoga can technically be practiced on any flat surface, it is beneficial to have a mat designed specially for yoga due to the following reasons:

1. Traction and Stability: A good yoga mat provides the necessary grip that keeps you from sliding during poses (like the Downward-Facing Dog).

2. Comfort: A mat cushions your body, reducing the direct impact on your knees, elbows, wrists, and other pressure points.

3. Hygiene: Having your own mat protects you from shared surfaces in public spaces.

When choosing a yoga mat, pay attention to the factors such as the material, thickness, size, texture, and eco-friendliness.

4.2. Yoga Props

Yoga props are designed to increase your comfort, balance, flexibility, and alignment while executing poses. They can be particularly helpful for beginners who might need assistance establishing correct form or stretching farther than their current ability allows. A well-equipped yoga kit should include the following props:

4.2.1. Yoga Blocks

Yoga blocks, usually made of foam, cork, or bamboo, are standard tools for boosting stability and flexibility. They are typically used in three different orientations, each providing a different level of support.

1. Standing Tall: The block offers maximum height for those who struggle to reach the ground in poses such as the Half Moon.

2. On Its Side: The medium height is beneficial for seated poses where one hand is on the ground for support.

3. Flat: Laying the block flat provides minimum height but maximum stability, great for restorative poses.

4.2.2. Yoga Straps

For beginner yogis who experience limited flexibility, a yoga strap can be a game-changer. Essentially extending your arms' reach, these straps allow you to perform poses that might otherwise be uncomfortable or impossible. They're particularly handy for poses requiring you to touch or hold your feet, such as the Seated Forward Bend or the Reclining Hand-to-Big-Toe Pose.

4.2.3. Yoga Bolsters

A yoga bolster is essentially a pillow designed for comfort and support in various yoga postures, often in restorative practices. They can be used to support the back in lying poses, provide cushioning in seated and kneeling positions, and even provide elevation in some poses.

4.2.4. Yoga Blankets

Yoga blankets offer extra padding, warmth, and support, making them a versatile prop. Folding and stacking yoga blankets can provide height and support to accommodate specific poses.

4.3. Yoga Attire

What you wear during your yoga practice can have a significant impact on your comfort and ease of movement. Look for clothing that is breathable, stretchable, and comfortable. It is usually best to wear form-fitting attire since loose clothing can get in the way during certain poses. Bear in mind that body temperature can vary throughout your practice, so layering can be a good option to stay comfortable during warm-up, main practice, and cooldown.

Remember, every yogi's journey is unique, and there is no one-size-fits-all approach when choosing your gear. The items mentioned in this guide serve as the foundation, but it's up to you to feel into what is necessary for your practice. Your gear will evolve as you do. As you deepen into your yoga journey, you might find yourself gravitating towards additional tools to support your evolving practice. Embrace the process and enjoy your journey step by step, breath by breath. Yoga is not just an exercise—it's a lifestyle, a transformation that begins within, and with the support of the right gear, it will manifest into a physical practice that uplifts and revives your being in wondrous ways. Welcome to your yoga journey, where the body, mind, and spirit unite in perfect harmony.

Chapter 5. Pose for the Camera: Mastering Basic Yoga Poses

Before you can flow seamlessly through an entire yoga sequence, it's crucial to first understand and perfect the most basic yoga poses, also known as asanas. These poses form the foundation of all yoga practices as they help you build strength, balance, flexibility, and focus.

5.1. Understanding Asanas

Asanas are physical postures that you adopt during yoga. There are multiple categories of asanas, including standing poses, seated poses, lying down poses, inverted poses, and twisting poses. Each of these categories stimulates your body in different ways and harbours distinct benefits.

The importance of understanding asanas comes from the fact that you need to perform them correctly to prevent injuries and truly experience their benefits. Let's start by understanding the essential yoga poses.

5.2. Mountain Pose (Tadasana)

One of the most basic yoga asanas, the mountain pose, is excellent for posture, stability, and calmness.

Follow these steps to perform Tadasana:

1. Stand tall with your feet hip-width apart. Your toes should be spread out, but your weight should be evenly distributed across

both feet.

2. Extend your spine upwards, lifting through the crown of your head, ensuring your shoulders are relaxed, and your palms are facing inwards.

3. Take deep, steady breaths and hold the posture for 30-60 seconds.

5.3. Downward Dog (Adho Mukha Svanasana)

Downward dog is a commonly practiced pose that stretches the entire body and offers a moment of rest during intense sequences.

To perform this asana, follow these steps:

1. Begin on your hands and knees with your wrists underneath your shoulders, and the knees underneath your hips.

2. Tuck your toes under and lift your hips up and back, straightening your legs.

3. Keep your arms straight, with your fingers spread wide and your gaze back towards your feet.

4. Stay in this pose for 1-3 minutes.

5.4. Cobra Pose (Bhujangasana)

The cobra pose is a beginner-friendly backbend that helps to strengthen the spine and stretch the chest, shoulders, and abdomen.

Bhujangasana can be performed this way:

1. Lie prone on the floor. Stretch your legs back with the tops of the feet on the floor.

2. Place your hands under your shoulders. Hug your elbows back

into your body.

3. On an inhale, begin to straighten your arms to lift your chest off
   the floor.

4. Hold the position for 15-30 seconds.

5.5. Warrior I (Virabhadrasana I)

Warrior I is part of the classic sequence known as Warrior poses. It strengthens the lower body while stretching the upper body.

Here's how to practice Warrior I:

1. Stand in Tadasana then step your feet about 4 feet apart.

2. Turn your right foot 90 degrees to the right and your left foot slightly to the right.

3. On an exhale, bend your right knee over the right ankle. Stretch up through your arms, lifting your rib cage away from your pelvis.

4. Stay in this pose for 30 seconds to 1 minute.

Chapter 6. Benefits of Basic Asanas

While each pose has its unique benefits, they all contribute to improving strength, flexibility, and balance in the body. They also help quiet the mind and create a connection between the body and the spirit.

For beginners, mastering these foundational yoga poses is crucial. They help you get comfortable on the mat, improve your body awareness, and prepare you to dive into complex sequences.

Chapter 7. Important Tips for Beginners

As a beginner, strive to learn and not to perfect the poses. Each body is different, and so is the range of motion. Use these tips to make your practice more comfortable.

- Warm-up before starting your yoga session. It prepares your body for the stretches and prevents injuries.

- Remember to breathe. Yoga is as much about breathing as it is about moving. Ensure your breath is calm and steady throughout your practice.

- Listen to your body. If something feels uncomfortable or painful, back out of the pose or adjust it to suit your body.

- Stay consistent. Practice regularly, even if it's a few minutes each day, to improve flexibility and comfort over time.

Yoga is a journey of self-discovery and body awareness. Embrace the process and enjoy the progress.

Chapter 8. Closing Note

The mastery of basic yoga poses forms the backbone of your yoga journey. As you learn to move through these poses with grace and ease, you'll be ready to take on more complex asanas and sequences. Remember, yoga is not about touching your toes, it is about what you learn about yourself on the way down. Start slow, be patient with your growth, and most importantly, enjoy the journey.

Chapter 9. Breathe Better: An Excursion into Pranayama

Pranayama, an integral part of yoga, is the science of breath control. It's a journey that comprises systematic techniques designed to gain mastery over the respiratory process while recognizing the connection between breath, mind, and emotions.

9.1. Roots of Pranayama

Before we delve deeper into the techniques and benefits of Pranayama, it's imperative to understand its roots. The word Pranayama can be broken down into two Sanskrit words - 'Prana' which is the vital energy or life force and 'Ayama' which implies control or extension. The exercise of Pranayama is rooted in the ancient yoga texts named the Upanishads and the Bhagavad Gita, which highlight the importance of controlling the breath to harness one's life energy.

9.2. Understanding the Breathing Dynamics

A journey into Pranayama begins with a simple act: observing the breath. On average, humans breathe about 20,000 times a day, often unconsciously. In contrast, Pranayama asks you to breathe consciously and mindfully. By observing your breath's rhythm, you begin to understand its connection to your mental and physical states. Rapid and irregular breaths are often associated with stress and anxiety, while slow, deep breaths often indicate a calm mind. Understanding breathing dynamics sets the foundation for proceeding further into the exploration of Pranayama.

9.3. Basic Breath Awareness

Technique	Description
Diaphragmatic Breathing	Most of us breathe from our chest, resulting in shallow breaths that don't fully oxygenate our bodies. Diaphragmatic breathing, or belly breathing, aims to reverse this pattern by retraining us to breathe from our abdomen. To practice, lie down on your back. Place one hand on your stomach and the other on your chest. As you breathe in, try to push the hand over your stomach up, while keeping the hand over your chest still. On exhaling, your belly should contract inward. Practising diaphragmatic breathing daily can lay the groundwork for deeper Pranayama practices.
4-7-8 Breathing	Renowned for its calming effect, the 4-7-8 breathing technique can pave the way for more advanced Pranayama exercises. It retrains the breathing pattern in a ratio of 4:7:8. Inhale through your nose for a count of 4, hold your breath for a count of 7, and then exhale through your mouth for a count of 8. Repeat this cycle at least four times to promote a relaxed state.

9.4. Pranayama Techniques

Technique	Description
Anulom Vilom	Known as Alternate Nostril Breathing, it brings balance and harmony by activating both brain hemispheres. Begin by sitting comfortably and closing your right nostril with your thumb, then inhale through your left nostril. Close the left nostril with your ring finger, open the right nostril and exhale through it. Inhale through the right nostril, close it, open the left nostril and exhale. Repeat the cycle for a few minutes.

Kapalbhat Kapalbhati, or "shining skull", involves short and
i   forceful exhalation followed by a passive inhalation. It's
             invigorating and can energize the mind and body. Start
             with a few rounds of diaphragmatic breathing. Then,
             take a comfortable deep inhale and expel the air
             forcefully by contracting your abdominal muscles. Allow
             inhalation to happen passively without any effort.
             Kapalbhati should be practiced under expert
             supervision, especially if you're a beginner.

9.5. Physiology of Pranayama

Pranayama can improve cardiovascular health, increase lung capacity and efficiency, enhance digestion, reduce stress, and aid in better sleep. Studies have suggested that regular Pranayama can improve autonomic functions by balancing the sympathetic and parasympathetic nervous systems, leading to increased mindfulness and a better mood.

9.6. Incorporating Pranayama into Daily Life

Incorporating Pranayama into your daily routine can be strategically beneficial for your physical and mental wellbeing. Whether you choose to start your day with a few rounds of Anulom Vilom or end your day with 4-7-8 breathing, the positive impact of a regulated breath can permeate your life. One suggestion is to link it with your existing habits – perform a few rounds of Pranayama after brushing your teeth or before your morning coffee.

9.7. Hungry for More?

Remember that yoga, including Pranayama, is a journey and not a destination. Feel free to explore, experiment and find what works best for you. Seek guidance from a knowledgeable teacher to ensure you're practicing safely. As you delve more deeply into this ancient art of breath control, you will uncover layers of peace, control, and vitality that can reshape your life.

In conclusion, mastering Pranayama is a lifelong journey. Just as a musical instrument brings forth the beauty of music only when one masters the nuances of playing it, the human body, too, reveals its full vitality when one learns to control and regulate one's breath.

Chapter 10. Mindful Movements: Exploring Yoga Flows and Sequences

Yoga, in its essence, is not just a set of static poses, but a dynamic exploration of movement and balance, often referred to as flow or "Vinyasa". Understanding and practicing these sequences allows us to move mindfully, intertwining breath and motion, physicality and mindfulness.

10.1. Breath and Movement: The Heart of Vinyasa

In Sanskrit, Vinyasa can be translated as "to place in a certain way," but it is often interpreted more freely as the connection between breath and movement. In Vinyasa yoga, each motion is carried out with an inhalation or an exhalation, creating a flow that mirrors the rhythmic pulsation of life itself.

Breath is your anchor throughout this practice. We begin and end every yoga session with focused breathing exercises. Learning to use your breath deliberately, and use it in conjunction with your movements, is vital. Start by taking a few moments to center yourself, sitting comfortably, and observing your natural breath. Over time, you'll develop a deep, steady Ujjayi breath, engaging your diaphragm, and filling and emptying your lungs fully.

10.2. The Sun Salutation: Your First Yoga Flow

Surya Namaskar, more commonly known as Sun Salutation, is the staple of many yoga practices. This sequence of poses is often used to begin a yoga session, whether in a studio class or in your personal practice. The Sun Salutation is not just a physical warm-up, but a way to pay homage to the interconnected physical and spiritual energies of the world.

A common variation of Surya Namaskar includes twelve poses:

1. Mountain Pose (Tadasana)

2. Upward Salute (Urdhva Hastasana)

3. Standing Forward Bend (Uttanasana)

4. Half Standing Forward Bend (Ardha Uttanasana)

5. Plank

6. Four-Limbed Staff Pose (Chaturanga Dandasana)

7. Cobra Pose (Bhujangasana)

8. Downward-Facing Dog (Adho Mukha Svanasana)

9. Half Standing Forward Bend (Ardha Uttanasana)

10. Standing Forward Bend (Uttanasana)

11. Upward Salute (Urdhva Hastasana)

12. Mountain Pose (Tadasana)

A complete round includes a second set, switching the leg that steps back into plank.

Each pose in this sequence is carried out with either an inhalation or an exhalation, thus creating the signature 'flow' of Vinyasa yoga. You'll weave these poses together into a graceful dance, powered by your breath. Over time, you'll come to know this flow well, feeling the gentle activation of every muscle in your body and growing more confident and competent in every pose.

10.3. Developing Your Own Sequences

Once you're comfortable with the Sun Salutation, you may want to explore creating your own sequences. The key to this is understanding the purpose and effect of each pose. Know your "peak pose" - the most challenging or specific posture you wish to work on for that day.

Choose a series of warm-up poses that prepare the body for this peak pose, stabilization poses that allow you to hold and deepen it, and finally some cool-down poses that allow for relaxation and integration of the benefits derived from the session.

10.4. The Importance of Savasana

No yoga session is complete without the final pose - Savasana, or "Corpse Pose". Despite its ominous name, it is a pose of relaxation and release. It allows for your body to integrate the physical and energetic shifts from your practice. This final resting pose allows you a moment to arrive back into stillness. The key to a deeply enriching Savasana lies not in the mere act of lying down, but in truly allowing yourself to release each muscle, each thought, surrendering completely to the pose, and to the present moment.

Remember that yoga is not about the perfect pose but the journey it took to get there. The movements, transitions, and breaths in between have as much importance as reaching the peak pose. Strive for consciousness more than perfection. Let your body guide you, let your breath sustain you and find joy in every movement. This is the perfect way to ensure a mindful and satisfying journey into yoga.

Chapter 11. Spicing Things Up: Exploring Various Yoga Styles

When stepping into the world of yoga, you might be surprised to discover just how many different styles there are. With the roots of yoga buried deep in ancient Indian philosophies, it's no wonder that over centuries, various practices have evolved, each with its own unique approach to achieving harmony of the mind-body-spirit triad. This chapter aims to dive deep into the vast ocean of yoga styles - some traditional, some modern, and some a fusion. Understanding these styles can help you identify which one aligns best with your disposition, lifestyle, and goals.

11.1. The Traditional Styles

[Traditional] Yoga Styles trace their roots back to ancient Indian traditions and texts. They focus heavily on spiritual and philosophical aspects apart from physical postures.

1. **Hatha Yoga**: Often considered the mother of all yoga styles, Hatha is the most traditional form of yoga. It involves a series of "asanas" (poses) accompanied by "pranayama" (breathing exercises). With slow-paced movements and a strong focus on breath, Hatha is perfect for beginners.

2. **Iyengar Yoga**: This style of yoga, named after its inventor B.K.S. Iyengar, emphasizes proper alignment in each pose. It stands unique for its use of props such as blocks, straps, and bolsters, making it accessible to individuals with varying levels of flexibility and strength.

3. **Ashtanga Yoga**: Intense and fast-paced, Ashtanga is a synchronized sequence of poses performed continuously.

Structured around six series, each with specific asanas, it's a challenging but rewarding style for those who appreciate a rigorous physical practice.

4. **Kundalini Yoga**: A blend of spiritual and physical practices, Kundalini yoga focuses on awakening the energy at the base of the spine. A typical class involves chanting, meditation, asanas, and breathwork.

11.2. The Modern Styles

[**Modern**] Yoga Styles have evolved predominantly in Western societies as a means to cater to contemporary requirements - focusing more on physical fitness and stress release.

1. **Vinyasa Yoga**: Descendant of Ashtanga, Vinyasa offers more flexibility regarding sequence structure. Each movement flows into the next with synchronicity to the breath, creating a "flow". It's popular for its dynamism and variation.

2. **Bikram Yoga**: Founded by Yogiraj Bikram Choudhury, this style features a fixed series of 26 postures and two breathing exercises - usually practiced in a hot room (around 40 °C). The heat promotes sweat, aiding in detoxification and flexibility.

3. **Power Yoga**: A vigorous fitness-based approach to yoga, Power Yoga is inspired by Ashtanga but has no fixed sequence. It focuses on building strength and often forgoes the spiritual aspects.

4. **Restorative Yoga**: As the name suggests, Restorative Yoga is about relaxation and healing. It uses props to support the body in restful positions, facilitating deep emotional and physical release.

11.3. Fusion Styles

[**Fusion**] Yoga Styles blend elements of yoga with other disciplines, creating innovative and integrated practices.

1. **Aerial Yoga**: This type blends traditional asanas with acrobatics, performed while suspended from silk hammocks. Ideal for those looking for a fun, unconventional workout.

2. **Yin Yoga**: A hybrid of Hatha and traditional Chinese medicine, Yin focuses on passive stretches held for longer durations. It targets the body's deep connective tissues, promoting the flow of 'qi' or life force.

3. **Yoga Nidra**: Also known as yogic sleep, it's a technique stemming from ancient Tantra practices. Guided meditations lead the practitioner into a state between wakefulness and sleep, providing profound relaxation.

Choosing a style doesn't confine you to its practice exclusively; explorative yogis often dabble across styles, finding value in the distinctive elements of each. A style that fits you today might not be what serves you tomorrow, and that's okay. The practice of yoga is, among many things, a journey of self-discovery. So, try different classes, meet with different teachers, and remember, the best style of yoga is the one that resonates with you and makes you show up on the mat, day after day. As your practice matures, you'll uncover the transformative power of yoga, not just on a physical level, but on a mental and spiritual one too. The world of yoga is waiting for you. Breathe deep... You're in for an amazing ride. Happy practicing!

Chapter 12. Nourish to Flourish: Integrating Yoga with Nutrition

Understanding the relationship between yoga and nutrition is key to establishing a comprehensive wellness routine. Recognizing their interconnection can lead to a richer, more holistic practice that uplifts both body and mind.

12.1. The Power of Food

Every morsel of food we ingest has an impact on our bodies, both immediately and in the long term. Eating the right nutrients at the right time can bring about a world of positive changes. We're not merely talking about feeling full after a meal - the food we choose to consume can affect everything from our mood, our energy level to our ability to concentrate. Achieving a state of well-being involves eating meals that enhance our physical capacity and mental clarity.

12.2. Sattvic, Rajasic, and Tamasic Food

The yogic dietary philosophy is based on the concept of Sattvic, Rajasic, and Tamasic foods. According to yogic tradition, these types of foods directly influence our consciousness and behavior.

Sattvic foods are believed to bring about clarity, understanding, and spiritual growth. These foods are easily digestible and beneficial to the body. They include fresh fruits, vegetables, nuts, seeds, and whole grains. These foods are typically grown organically and consumed in as natural a state as possible - fresh, raw, and minimally processed.

Rajasic foods are thought to incite passion, ego, and restlessness. They include dry, spicy, salty, and bitter foods, such as coffee, tea, and processed food.

Tamasic foods are associated with ignorance, doubt, and pessimism. These foods are generally processed, overcooked, stale, or fermented, like alcohol, fried foods, and re-heated leftovers.

A yoga-focused diet would prioritize Sattvic foods while minimizing Rajasic and Tamasic items for optimal health and mental clarity.

12.3. Yoga and Digestion

Unlike other forms of physical exercise, yoga asanas are not just about building strength or flexibility. They are about harmonizing the body's internal processes too. Specific yoga asanas can stimulate digestive health, improve metabolism, and enhance nutrient absorption. Paired with a wholesome, nutritious diet, these asanas can bring about significantly improved digestive wellbeing.

Consider incorporating asanas like the 'Pawanmuktasana' (Wind-Relieving Pose) or 'Ardha Matsyendrasana' (Half Spinal Twist) in your routine to stimulate gut motility and digestion.

12.4. Hydration and Yoga

Hydration is crucial for any physical activity, and yoga is no exception. While we often attribute sweating and vigorous movement to water loss and hydration needs, the less visible physiological processes are equally, if not more, important. Our body requires water for countless internal processes, so maintain regular and substantial water intake.

12.5. Mindful Eating

In the context of yoga, eating isn't just about what you eat, but also how you eat. Practicing mindfulness can be hugely beneficial in your eating habits. Take a moment before your meal to appreciate the food, chew slowly, and savor every mouthful. Mindful eating can significantly influence digestion, nutrient absorption, and overall health.

It's important to remember that yoga doesn't begin and end on the mat - it's a lifestyle. Provoking thoughtfulness about the foods you eat and integrating wholesome, nutritious choices into your routine is a step towards a truly yogic lifestyle.

12.6. Planning A Yoga Diet

In practical terms, how can all of this wisdom be condensed into your daily routine? How do you go about planning meals keeping in mind the yogic principles and nutritional needs? Here are a few tips: - Begin by gradually introducing more Sattvic foods into your diet. - Replace processed snacks with fresh fruits, nuts, and seeds. - Reduce the intake of stimulants like caffeine and processed sugar. - Prepare meals using fresh ingredients and minimize the use of canned or prepackaged foods. - Set regular meal times to maintain a consistent digestive rhythm.

Aside from these steps, it is crucial to listen to your body. Yoga encourages us to develop a heightened sense of awareness about our bodies. So observe the effects different foods have on your body and mind.

Remember, integrating yoga with nutrition isn't about deprivation or strict dieting. It's about nourishing your body with foods that uplift you both physically and mentally, fostering a sense of overall well-being. While this might feel overwhelming at first, small consistent changes can gradually lead to a significant overall improvement. As with yoga, the key to dietary changes is patience and persistence.

In conclusion, yoga and nutrition share a harmonious relationship, the understanding and practice of which can lead to a holistically fulfilling life experience. By integrating both into your life, you can create a lifestyle that supports not only physical health but also overall mental and spiritual well-being. Nourish to flourish indeed.

Chapter 13. Riding the Wave: Overcoming Challenges in Yoga

Diving deep into any new practice often comes with its fair share of trials and challenges. Yoga, while offering a multitude of healing and self-realization benefits, is no different. The road may not always be smooth, and you will find yourself facing barriers of both physical and mental nature. However, these barriers are not your enemies; they are catalysts for growth, helping you find strength and resilience you never knew you had.

13.1. Understanding the Challenges

Many beginners view yoga as a simple sequence of physical movements. In reality, it's an intricate balance of mind and body, breath, and spirit, which can sometimes be overwhelming. Understanding the nature of the challenges you may encounter is the first step in overcoming them.

13.1.1. The Physical Hurdle

Like any other physical activity, yoga brings about muscular exertion. General fatigue, muscle soreness, lack of flexibility, and difficulty in perfecting asanas can pose significant challenges to beginners. This hurdle becomes overwhelmingly noticeable particularly when advancing from simple to more complex poses.

13.1.2. The Mental Struggle

Yoga also necessitates mental strength and discipline. Patience, focus, determination, and commitment are vital elements of this practice.

Without these, achieving your desired level of peace and self-awareness can be a tough road to navigate.

13.1.3. The Breath Control Test

Pranayama, or breath control, is an essential component of yoga, and it has profound effects on your mind and body. However, for novices, mastering controlled breathing can be particularly challenging. Balancing physical movements while controlling the breathing rhythm requires patience, practice, and depth of understanding about how your body meshes with your breath.

13.2. Building Resiliency Through Yoga

Yoga is not just about overcoming challenges but also about learning and blossoming through them. The hurdles faced during yoga are stepping stones that build your resilience and transform you inside out.

13.2.1. The Power of Consistency

The secret to overcoming the physical hurdle lies in consistency. Regular practice creates flexibility and strength, making asanas easier over time. The body has a remarkable ability to adapt, but it requires dedication and persistence.

13.2.2. The Beauty of Patience and Focus

Cultivating mental strength can take time – patience is key. Simultaneously, keeping your focus sharp enables a deeper engagement with the practice. Meditative components of yoga, such as Dhyana or meditation, could immensely help in training your mind.

13.2.3. Mastering Your Breath

Pranayama, when practiced regularly, becomes a natural part of your yoga routine. It can slowly teach you that the breath is not just a means to live, but a powerful tool for balance and control.

13.3. Overcoming Commonly Faced Challenges

Addressing some of the most commonly faced challenges by novices effectively.

13.3.1. Stage of Comparison

In the beginning, it's normal to compare your progress with others. However, each body is different, and progress comes at its unique pace. Embrace your journey, celebrate small victories and slowly, you will notice progress.

13.3.2. Lack of Time

Despite the popular belief, yoga does not require numerous hours of dedication daily. Even twenty minutes of daily practice can yield magnificent results over time. It's about quality, not quantity.

13.3.3. Overwhelm of Technical Terms

Yoga, with its roots in ancient India, is laden with Sanskrit terms. However, don't let this be a point of stress. With time and regular involvement, these will become familiar, much like any other language you'd acquire.

Conclusively, the journey of yoga is unique for every individual. The challenges are opportunities to break through self-imposed limitations and reveal your innate power. Embrace every twist, every stretch, every breath - and remember; every moment of struggle is a moment of growth. Let the wave of challenges wash over you - they're not here to swamp you but to lift you higher into the realm of self-realization.

Chapter 14. A Lifetime of Wellness: Maintaining Your Yoga Practice

Maintaining your yoga practice over the long term requires a fusion of commitment, versatility, strategies for motivation and a deep understanding of the many dimensions that constitute 'Yoga'. This awareness ensures that your yoga journey continues to grow, and does not stagnate over time.

14.1. Approach, Set Goals, but Be Flexible

A consistent yoga practice requires a realistic and flexible approach. Set achievable goals for yourself, such as attending a yoga class two to three times per week or setting aside specific times for your home practice. But remember, flexibility is key. If a conflict arises and you miss a class, don't let it throw you off. Just make sure you return to the mat the next day.

Don't pressure yourself to execute the perfect version of a pose right away. Every body is different, and poses will look different for everyone. Yoga isn't a competitive sport, but it's rather an integral pathway to wellness, self-discovery, and peace. Patience, practice, and time will naturally deepen and evolve your practice.

14.2. Enrich Your Practice with Diverse Styles

Incorporating different styles of yoga into your routine will not only keep your practice interesting, but it will also help you develop a more rounded skill set. Experiment with styles like Hatha, Ashtanga, Iyengar, Kundalini, Vinyasa, Yin, and Restorative.

Each of these styles contributes distinct benefits to your mental and physical wellbeing. Hatha improves flexibility and reduces stress, Ashtanga increases strength and stamina, Iyengar focuses on the alignment, Kundalini uplifts your spiritual wellbeing, Vinyasa enhances breathing efficiency, Yin is great for deep tissue mobility and Restorative facilitates deep relaxation and balance.

14.3. Keep the Equipment Handy

Having the right gear is essential to help cultivate a sustained yoga routine. Invest in a good quality mat that provides you with enough grip and cushioning. Other useful yoga tools that support your practice include yoga blocks, straps, bolster pillows, and blankets. While these may not be necessary at the onset, they can significantly enhance your practice as you progress.

14.4. Cultivating Mind-Body Harmony

Yoga cannot be reduced to just asanas or poses. It is also about forging that precious mind-body connection which can bring transformative changes to your life beyond the yoga mat. Practice mindfulness during your session, focusing on your body, the movements, and your breath.

Integrating Pranayama or conscious breathing techniques into your practice can elevate this sense of connection. Pranayama exercises like Anulom Vilom (alternate nostril breathing), Ujjayi (victorious breath), and Kapalabhati (skull shining breath) can help to clear mental fog, improve respiratory health, and build inner fire.

14.5. Healing Yourself with Yoga Philosophy

Immerse yourself in the eight limbs of yoga as introduced in Patanjali's Yoga Sutras, a foundational text in yoga philosophy. The eight limbs - Yama (ethical principles), Niyama (spiritual observances), Asana (posture), Pranayama (breath control), Pratyahara (withdrawal of the senses), Dharana (concentration), Dhyana (meditative absorption), and Samadhi (bliss) – serve as guidance on how to lead a meaningful and purposeful life.

Understanding and integrating these principles make you more introspective, helping to handle life's up and downs with equanimity and grace. You'll find that yoga becomes less an 'exercise' and more a 'way of life'.

14.6. Connecting with the Yoga Community

Bonding with a community, whether online or offline, can greatly nourish your motivation to maintain your yoga practice. Join local, invigorating yoga classes, attend workshops, retreats, or festivals. Online yoga communities also offer ample opportunities for learning and connection. You can share your yoga journey, get inspired by fellow practitioners, and always find encouragement and support, which is very much essential in sustaining your practice.

14.7. Listen to Your Body

Respecting the body's signals is crucial in maintaining a long-term yoga practice. Differentiate between the good pain that comes with stretching and challenging your body and the sharp, bad pain of injury. Don't force a pose. Instead, ease into it. With time, your flexibility will improve, and you'll be more capable of doing the pose without risk.

14.8. Sustainability is Key

Remember, yoga is not a sprint but a marathon. The best way to maintain your long-term yoga practice is by staying committed, yet flexible, honoring your body, learning continuously, and celebrating your journey. The destination is important, but yoga teaches us to be present and to enjoy the journey as we get there. So, find joy in each breath, each pose, each challenge, and every achievement in your practice.

And most importantly, remember that yoga is a tool for self-care, self-discovery, and personal growth. The mat is your sacred space – a place for you to come back to, again and again, to recenter, refocus, and rejuvenate. Whether you are a beginner starting your journey, or an experienced practitioner, letting the principles of yoga seep into your life on and off the mat, will pave the path for a healthier, happier, and harmonious life.